Spices to the Rescue

by

Hanna Kroeger

Copyright

Table of Contents

Section I: Spices

Section II:
Additional Kitchen Remedies

Spices to the Rescue
by Hanna Kroeger

Introduction

Food and spices have always been an important part of life and in many ways define a culture. Garlic and oregano are undeniably Italian, ginger and chop sticks are good friends, and turmeric and sitar music are a natural. Great explorations brought new spices and foods to and from Europe, Asia, Africa, and the Americas. Philosophers would pontificate the virtues of a particular spice and the value of spices and foods were realized in everyday life.

Spices to the Rescue is first aid from your kitchen. The suggestions are very practical for everyday use, the kind of advice your grandmother would give you. It includes easy preparations and recommendations for using spices and foods to help with everyday health. You will want to keep this book in the kitchen near your spices.

We know these spices for their culinary beauty, now we get to discover the beauty of their health virtues. *Spices to the Rescue* contains interesting insight into the time proven historical uses of spices and how they can become a valuable part of your health.

Section I: Spices

~ Alfalfa Seed ~

Alfalfa seeds are loaded with vitamin C. Alfalfa contains many trace minerals and, when used as a tea, releases pain in the head and limbs. If you sprout alfalfa seeds and eat 2 tablespoons of sprouts twice a day, it will lower cholesterol. Alfalfa stimulates the appetite and improves digestion. It is a very good mineral supplier and helps make the bowels move. Alfalfa is a good source of vitamin K. Alfalfa sprouts will help rid the body of excess cholesterol. ~

~ Allspice ~

Allspice can be used if couples are inharmonious. It is also very effective if you are inharmonious with yourself. It is balm to the liver. It is known to relieve colic and gas. Boil the crushed fruit and apply on a cloth to aid rheumatism and neuralgia.

For general use, you can chew three kernels twice a day. If parts of the body are hot or cold, or a condition can be called "one sided neuralgia" or you have a one sided headache, take 1/2 teaspoon crushed allspice in juice twice a day. ~

~ **Anise** ~

This delicate, feathery spice has been used medicinally for centuries. In 1500 B.C., the Egyptians grew great quantities of anise for use in food, drink, and medicine. Early colonists carried anise seeds to North America where it was grown as a medicinal spice.

What a blessing is anise. Make a tea for indigestion and for the three months of colic that so many babies suffer from. It is also excellent to soothe the stomach after vomiting and works well on a bloated stomach which can result in headaches. It is particularly effective for bloatedness in babies.

Old asthmatic cases love anise tea and it has been found to be useful for relieving asthma. Numbness in the lower lip is remedied by a sprinkle of anise or anise tea.

In olden times, anise was used to heal kidney stones. They put 1 tablespoon of anise in 1 quart of grape juice and simmered it for 1/2 hour. They drank 7 ounces 3 times a day. Anise oil was also used to relieve jaundice.

Ten to 12 drops of anise oil in 1 tablespoon of warm water improves liver functioning. Anise also helps when people have unpleasant breath.

Anise is a comforting antiseptic tea for colds and coughs. It can help bronchial problems. It is useful for gas and as a diuretic when used with caraway and fennel. Anise tea helps relieve hiccups.

Anise is used for a bloated condition, especially in infants. It has been used to enhance the milk production in nursing mothers. Anise and caraway tea remove poisons by flushing them out.

It can be added to laxative formulas to prevent cramping of the bowels. It is useful for breaking up mucous and for dry, hard coughs.

~ Basil ~

Basil was said to have been found growing around Christ's tomb after the resurrection, and some churches use basil to prepare holy water while others set it around their alters. The Indians swore their oaths upon this herb.

In some cultures, it is carried in the pocket to magnetize money. Its aromatic influence is said to help one to have an open mind.

Basil is food for the brain. When you feel victimized or criticized, eat some basil. If you wash your hands, arms, and face with basil tea, you can cope with an unfriendly world better. It is an antidepressant and is helpful for nervous exhaustion and mental fatigue. It is known to stimulate the adrenal cortex.

Basil is an excellent anti-viral spice and is used for colds, flu, chills, nausea, and to prevent vomiting. It is used for indigestion, kidney and bladder troubles, headaches, cramps, and constipation. A tea made of 1 ounce basil simmered in 1 pint of water for 20 minutes with 6 powdered black peppercorns will relieve most fevers.

Basil is an insect repellent and the juice is used for snake bites in India. Applied to the skin, it is useful to relieve itching and ringworm.

～ Bay Leaf ～

In Roman history, bay leaves were used for prophecy and healing. A wreath of bay leaves became the mark of excellence for poets and athletes and a symbol of wisdom and glory. It was used against plagues for many centuries.

Bay leaf is a digestive aid and stimulates the appetite. Massaging bay leaf oil around sprains and into rheumatic joints can bring relief. It is a natural insect repellent and is used in potpourri to repel insects, as well as for its simple beauty and aroma.

When bay leaves are combined with cinnamon, sage, and cloves and boiled in apple juice, they make an excellent natural cold remedy. ⤸

~ **Black Pepper** ~

Black Pepper is thought to be one of nature's most perfect foods, as it both cures and prevents many diseases. It kills bacteria and can be used as a food preservative.

It is a digestive aid, relieving gas, and has been used as a tea for running bowels. It is good for constipation, nausea, vertigo, and arthritis.

It is a diuretic and a stimulant. Black pepper is loaded with chromium which is needed for the proper functioning of the pancreas and heart.

For an earache, oil a piece of cotton and sprinkle it with freshly ground black pepper. Place it over the ear, *not in the ear canal.* For sinus problems or an infection in the sinuses, take 1 teaspoon of honey, sprinkle with freshly ground black pepper and eat it. ⤸

~ **Black Tea** ~

Used as part of everyday life, black tea is also a powerful medicinal herb. The Chinese have been using this herb for thousands of years to promote good health. It is a stimulant and digestive aid and is now known to prevent stomach and skin cancers.

Black tea reduces high blood pressure, lowers cholesterol, and reduces the risk of arterial disease. Rich in natural fluoride, it reduces tooth decay. A wet tea bag applied to an insect sting has been found to bring quick relief. It has been used for diarrhea, food poisoning, and hangovers.

In the hospital in Turkey, when a person was badly burned, we made a quart of black tea and poured it over the burn again and again. They healed very quickly. Drinking black tea is also helpful for the relief of sore and tender ovaries.

~ **Borage** ~

"I, borage, always bring courage." John Gerard, 1597, quoting the old Latin adage, *ergo borago gaudia semper ago.*

Borage has been used throughout history to comfort the heart, dispel depression, and give courage. This marvelous cooking herb stimulates the adrenal glands, where courage begins, and enhances the body's production of adrenaline.

The delicate, slightly sweet blue flowers were used by the Old Masters to color the paint used for the Madonna's robe. It has been added to salads for hundreds of years to "make the mind glad."

Borage promotes sweating and lactation and can be used for depression, grief, and anxiety. A tea made from the leaves has been found to reduce dry, rasping coughs. The oil extracted from the seeds is available in capsules and is used for menstrual problems, rheumatic disorders, and applied to the skin for eczema and other rashes or dry skin.

Borage has been used for irritable bowel syndrome and for the relief of a hangover. It is also thought to be helpful when taken as a tincture for stress and as a tonic following steroid therapy.

~ Caraway ~

Caraway has a long history of use. It has been found in the remains of Stone Age meals, in Egyptian tombs, and along the ancient resting places of the Silk Road in Asia.

Caraway is very much like anise and, when mixed with anise, is twice as good. It is antispasmodic, improves the appetite, and subsides gastric distention. It is a digestive aid, is used for colic and nervous conditions, and prevents cramping when added to a laxative formula. It helps relieve phlegm and sweetens the breath.

To increase mothers milk, take 1 teaspoon of caraway seeds and put in 8 ounces of cold water. Bring to a boil and simmer for a few minutes. Drink several cups a day.

To use as a diuretic, take equal parts of caraway, fennel, and anise (about 1 teaspoon of each) and add to 1 pint of water. Bring to a boil and simmer for 15 minutes. Drink this amount twice a day.

– **Cardamom** –

Cardamom is an eye and brain food and should be used much more frequently than we use it. It has a soothing effect on all membranes, including the stomach and lungs. As a tea used for fever, use equal parts of cardamom and cloves.

Cardamom is commonly used to treat indigestion and gas. It warms and stimulates the body. Cardamom is used for colic, diarrhea, and headaches.

Some people cannot digest bananas. After eating bananas, chew a few cardamom seeds and the indigestion caused by bananas will be alleviated.

The skin of cardamom which is usually discarded can be burnt into ash. Six to 12 grains of this ash, when combined with honey and water, subsides vomiting.

~ Cayenne Pepper ~

Cayenne originated in Central and South America where it was used by the natives for many diseases, especially diarrhea and cramps. Cayenne was first introduced to the Western culture in 1548, coming from India.

It is a superior crisis spice, useful for many conditions. It is a stimulant to the entire body and has been used medicinally to warm the body and alleviate depression, chills, and rheumatism. It stimulates circulation and sweating and, when used topically, it is a counterirritant and brings circulation to an area. *(Do not use on broken skin.)*

Cayenne benefits the heart and prevents heart attacks, strokes, colds, and the flu. It improves overall vitality and is not irritating to the system when uncooked. When taken in capsules, cayenne probably treats cardiovascular disease by acting as a stimulant and reducing cholesterol buildup. It binds bile and cholesterol in the intestinal tract, which is then excreted.

Cayenne also aids in the relief of gastric ulcers, depression, chronic fatigue, and prostration. Drinking cayenne pepper in cream is used to treat electrical shock. When there is pain from the hips to the feet take 1 cup of hot water with cayenne in it.

Cayenne can be rubbed on a toothache and used for swelling and inflammation. When cayenne tincture is rubbed on an arthritic joint and wrapped with flannel cloth overnight, the pain is usually gone by morning.

Cayenne normalizes circulation and can be used to stop bleeding, as well as for either high or low blood pressure. It is also helpful when there is shivering after drinking.

When used as a poultice, cayenne helps draw out impurities imbedded in flesh. It stimulates the nervous system and the digestive system. It is antibacterial and has been found to be helpful for sore throats, colds, laryngitis, hoarseness, and chills.

Cayenne is indicated when the ears are stinging or burning, when there is swelling behind the ears, or for Eustachian tube difficulties. If the ears are burning, drink cayenne in a little hot water. If there is a swelling behind the ear, put cayenne in a little water and rub on the back of the ear.

For aching feet, sprinkle cayenne in the socks. Hot peppers and radishes contain benzene which

is needed for proper functioning of the feet and sinuses. Cayenne, when eaten in food, can relieve
homesickness or the need to be alone.

*Do not use the seeds, as they can be toxic, and
do not touch the eyes or open sores after touching
cayenne pepper or chilies.*

– Celery –

Celery is both an important food and medicinal
spice. It has been used in the spring as a tonic to
clear out the stagnation of winter toxins. It is a
mild sedative and is restorative for weak conditions.

Celery increases uric acid excretion. It has
been used as a kidney cleanser and for the re-
moval of urinary stones. For kidney and bladder
troubles, eat celery tops after each meal for 5
weeks.

Celery aids in protein digestion. It increases
appetite and is useful in mucous conditions. It is
used in gastric troubles, colds, and coughs.

Celery has been found to be beneficial for respiratory ailments. Eating fresh stalks of celery after childbirth can stimulate milk production. Celery juice is very helpful for joint inflammation,
rheumatoid arthritis, and nervous exhaustion.

~ **Cinnamon** ~

The use of cinnamon goes back to ancient history. It is said that King Solomon recommended its use and it was used freely by the Arabs, Phoenicians, Greeks, and Romans. This delightful spice has been used throughout history to warm the body. It has a calming effect and is said to have a frequency which attracts wealth.

Cinnamon is used for fighting viral and infectious diseases. Virus, bacteria, and fungus cannot live in the presence of cinnamon oil. It is helpful for chills, colds, and arthritis.

Cinnamon can be used as an aid to digestive processes and alleviates indigestion, diarrhea, cramps, gas, and colic. It has been used for nausea and vomiting.

Cinnamon is warming and energizing to the kidneys. It has been found to be helpful for asthma, wheezing, and coughing. Certain pains have been known to respond to cinnamon such as lower back pain, abdominal pain, and heart pain.

Cinnamon is useful for menopausal difficulties and scanty menses.

It is a germicide, blood conditioner, and helps circulation. For children, cinnamon is useful to alleviate bed-wetting and to help them sleep.

Bleeding bowels:
   One half cup cinnamon tea 4 times a day or
   chew on cinnamon bark until you can visit
   your physician.

To remove fallout, radiation, or lead poisoning
from the system:
   Toast 1 slice of bread very brown. Butter it and
   sprinkle cinnamon on it. You can also add
   brown sugar or honey.

For colds:
   Combine cinnamon, sage, bay leaves, and
   cloves and boil in apple juice.

~ **Cloves** ~

Cloves are also called Peruvian Balm. Truly it
is a balm if you have bronchial catarrh or other
loud rattles in the chest. If you suffer from mucous in the chest or urine, cloves will benefit your
condition. Take 1 cup of hot water and add a
dash of cloves. If you want to add some honey,
that is fine. This recipe will also help relieve nausea and vomiting. If you suffer from eczema with
ulceration, drink 3 cups of clove water a day.

Cloves are used for anorexia, chronic cold, abdominal upset and gastric difficulties. It acts as a
breath freshener when chewed. It subsides gas
and expels worms.

Cloves are beneficial to the liver when it is swollen and hard, damaged, or contains tumors. Cloves in your tea will heighten your memory and a tea made of equal parts of cloves and cardamom is used for fever.

To use cloves to relieve a toothache, insert a little oil of cloves in the cavity or roll a bruised clove around in the mouth. To make oil of cloves, take a handful of cloves, bruise them, pack them into a jar, and cover with olive oil until the jar is full. Strain the oil after one week, save the oil, and add fresh cloves. This can be repeated as often as necessary until the oil is saturated with cloves.

Clove concentrate can be made in the following way: bruise a handful of cloves, steep in boiling water, then simmer for a few minutes. Do not allow the water to be reduced too much or it will be too strong. One teaspoon of this mixture added to 1 cup of hot water will make a tea which has a soothing, slightly sedative effect.

This tea can also be used for depression. It is said that the aroma of clove tea will create a feeling of protection and courage.

For a paper cut on the finger, wet the finger and dip it into powdered cloves. The pain quickly disappears because of clove's anesthetic effect on the skin.

~ **Coriander** ~

Coriander has been cultivated for over 3,000 years and is mentioned in the Bible where it is compared to manna. Coriander was brought to Europe by the Romans, who used it as a preservative for meat. The Chinese once believed it gave immortality.

Coriander is a digestive tonic and mild sedative. As an oil, it can be rubbed on painful and rheumatic joints. It is cooling, soothing, and calming to the body. It relieves fever when used as a tea. It is also helpful for gas and indigestion.

~ **Dill** ~

"Woe unto you, scribes, and Pharisees, hypocrites! for ye pay tithe of mint and dill and cumin, and have omitted the weightier matters of the law." (Matthew 23:23)

This Bible verse indicates that herbs such as dill were once so valued that they could be used to pay taxes.

Dill is widely used in the kitchen in sauces and to season cucumbers, vegetables, and potatoes. Dill also has many healing properties, particularly the seed.

The word "dill" comes from the Saxon word "to lull" because it has many tranquilizing effects. Dill is very useful for its high natural mineral salt content.

Dill Tea:
1 teaspoon dill seeds to 8 ounces cold water. Bring to a boil. Simmer for 10 minutes. Drink before or with a meal.

Dill tea helps relieve gas, indigestion, cramps, and colic. It has been used for hiccups and insomnia and it increases mothers milk. The seeds can be chewed to freshen breath.

Simmer dill seeds in olive oil and rub this oil on the forehead for better sleeping. Rubbing this oil on the abdomen takes pain away, eases infection, and relieves liver trouble and hardened conditions. The oil is also recommended for hemorrhoids and painful fissures.

To overcome hardened bowel movements, simmer 1 teaspoon of dill seed in 1 cup of boiling water, strain, and eat the hot seeds on bread. Drink the remaining tea for improvement of digestive processes.

Additionally, dill seeds and alfalfa seeds are thought to be beneficial to slow-learning children.

~ **Fennel** ~

"So gladiators fierce and rude
mingled it with their daily food.
And he who battled and subdued
a wreath of Fennel wore."
(Henry Wadsworth Longfellow)

Fennel is one of the oldest cultivated plants and was highly valued by the Romans. The warriors used it to maintain good health and the women ate it to prevent obesity. Chewing fennel seeds relieves hunger and eases digestion. It is delicious and naturally sweet.

Used as a mouthwash, fennel is thought to help loose teeth, gum disorders, laryngitis, and sore throats. Its aromatic influences increase longevity, courage, and purification.

Fennel Tea:
Simmer 1 teaspoon fennel seeds in 1 cup of water for 10 minutes. Drink 3 to 4 cups daily to balance obese condition. Additionally, fennel seeds can be added to salads to ease this condition. This tea is also excellent in conditions of cold and flu.

Fennel as a medicine to relieve colic conditions:
Add 1 teaspoon fennel seeds to 1 cup of water. Bring to a boil and simmer for 10 minutes. Strain and give children 1 teaspoon in water

every hour, adults 2 tablespoons in water every hour.

When a nursing mother drinks fennel tea, it promotes lactation and can relieve colic in the nursing child. It is helpful in reproductive system difficulties and the tea is an old folk remedy to regulate difficult and irregular menstrual periods. It has a hormonal - like action that reduces the effect of PMS and menopausal symptoms. Use fennel tea up to 3 times a day before and during the period.

To promote the free flow of urine, combine fennel seeds with caraway seeds and juniper and drink the tea.

Fennel in food will help digestion greatly. Too much stomach acidity can be regulated by taking 1 cup of fennel tea. Fennel expels mucous and relieves colic, cramps, bloated condition, gas, and constipation. It is beneficial to the kidneys and spleen and helps in urinary tract problems.

It can be used as an eyewash (make a tea, strain it, and bathe your eyes with it) and it has been used throughout history to improve eyesight. It is good for chronic coughs and other respiratory complaints. It is a circulatory stimulant. Make the tea, strain, and put in the bath to detoxify the body and release toxic waste. This can also be helpful in a hangover situation.

Fennel oil displays the same health-giving properties as the tea. ≈

~ **Fenugreek** ~

Fenugreek is one of the oldest medicinal plants and is a versatile spice. The Egyptians valued fenugreek for eating, healing, and embalming. It is useful for lung congestion and mucous conditions.

Fenugreek is helpful in relieving ulcers and other inflamed conditions of the stomach and intestines. It relieves fever, diarrhea, and gas. It is used in the treatment of diabetes and gout and is an excellent tonic and rejuvenator.

Used as a poultice of hot milk and crushed seeds, fenugreek relieves inflammation, swollen glands, sciatica, and bruises. ≈

~ **Flax** ~

Flax has been cultivated since at least 5000 B.C. In 8th century France, Charlemagne required his subjects to consume the seeds so they would remain healthy. Today, flax is still used as a bulk food in laxatives. It is also helpful for sore throats, bronchitis, hoarseness, and coughs. A tea made from the seeds is thought to help pulmonary infections.

Flax seed contains a remarkable healing oil which can be used externally or internally. Flax oil is useful for eczema, arthritis, menstrual cramps, and atherosclerosis. It has also been found to be beneficial to sprains and simple tumors. ≈

~ **Garlic** ~

Garlic has been prized by healers for more than 5,000 years. Pyramid builders and Roman soldiers on long marches were given a daily ration of garlic. Garlic is so strong an antibiotic that the English purchased tons of it during World War I for use on wounds. Journals of that period state that, when garlic was used on wounds, there were no cases of sepsis. It is a world renowned cure-all and home remedy in practically every culture. Today, even orthodox medicine accepts its healing powers.

Garlic has properties which help both the physical and mental bodies. When feeling discouraged, and negative thoughts are taking your happiness, burn garlic skin (that dry skin you throw away when peeling the garlic) slowly on an incense burner and the results are immediate. It also quiets the body and can be used as a mild tranquilizer.

Garlic contains selenium in a natural form, which is an antidote to mercury poisoning. It contains natural antibiotics and is known as the poor man's penicillin. While garlic only has 1 percent of the impact of penicillin, it is more effective than penicillin with gram negative bacteria.

Garlic sweeps through the body as a natural cleanser and tonic with no side effects. It maintains a healing factor in the bloodstream for up to 10 hours and doesn't destroy the body's friendly bacteria.

Garlic has properties which are anti-fungal, antibiotic, and anti-viral. It is a stimulant to the immune system, prevents colds and other illnesses, and has been used to treat mononucleosis and staph. It is used for coughs and bronchial congestion. It is an extremely important addition to any diet.

Garlic is an excellent remedy for long-term cardiovascular difficulties. It reduces blood cholesterol, strengthens arteries, and reduces the risk of further heart attacks in people who have already suffered one heart attack.

Garlic regulates blood pressure (so it is used for both high and low blood pressure) and it is an anticoagulant, which means it may prevent strokes. It helps unclog arteries coated with plaque and is an aid in combatting hypertension. Garlic helps regulate blood sugar levels and is known to be beneficial in cases of adult onset diabetes.

You can prepare garlic oil in the following way:
Take 1/2 pound of peeled and crushed garlic cloves. Put in a jar and cover with olive oil. Close tightly and shake a few times each day for 3 days, storing in a warm place. Strain through a clean cotton cloth. Store this garlic oil in a cool place.

For an earache, drop a little garlic oil into the ear. Leave it for only 10 minutes and then remove it with some cotton. For flu or colds, take 1 teaspoon of the oil every hour.

Garlic is anti-parasitic and helps the body rid itself of worms and other parasites. The recipe for using garlic to get rid of worms is as follows:
Cut 3 cloves of garlic. Boil in 1 cup of milk for 5 minutes. Let it cool enough to drink and strain. Drink this "Garlic Milk" every night for 10 nights in a row.

It is also useful in digestive disorders such as gastroenteritis and dysentery. Garlic has been found to block the formation of colon cancer and may prevent many other cancers.

Used fresh on the skin, garlic has been known to heal acne and other skin problems. Rubbing raw garlic on warts and corns is said to heal them. It promotes sweating and acts like an antihistamine. Rubbing garlic directly on an insect sting relieves the pain.

If garlic weren't so cheap, we would treasure it as much as pure gold. ⌐

– **Gentian** –

Gentian is a fabulous tonic. If your stomach feels full and bloated, 1/2 to 1 cup of gentian tea will do wonders. It is for colic and bloated conditions.

If your brain feels fuzzy, your head is tender, and your eyes hurt, gentian tea will relieve your difficulties. Gentian is also helpful for food poisoning. Gentian alleviates fevers, cools the body, and maintains digestive functions during a fever to prevent the stagnation of food.

Chewing gentian root has been known to help break the habit of smoking. ⌐

– **Ginger** –

". . . it is profitable for the stomach"
                              John Gerard 1597

Ginger is a blessing to an upset stomach. A pinch of ginger (about 1/4 teaspoon) to about 6 ounces of hot water is sufficient to bring relief. Ginger has long been known for its soothing effect to the stomach and has frequently been added to other herbs to act as a buffer in the stomach.

Ginger has been used as a medicine for thousands of years. It promotes sweating and reduces nausea and gas. It is an excellent stimulant for both the circulatory system and the immune system. It has been used for digestive disorders and urinary difficulties. It is also effective for travel sickness and sickness in pregnancy.

To make Ginger tea:
Use 1 to 2 teaspoons of granulated Jamaican ginger to 2 cups of boiling water. Pour the hot water over the ginger. Cover the container and allow the tea to steep until sufficiently cool to drink. Drink 1/2 to 1 cup at a time. Ginger tea may be flavored with a few cloves or a dash of nutmeg.

Hot compresses of ginger tea on the stomach will relieve cramping. It is helpful for stomach flu, both as a tea to drink and a compress on the stomach.

Ginger tea is also indicated for confusion, debility, and cramps in soles of feet or palms of hands. When joints feel weak or there is a heavy feeling in the stomach, ginger tea will bring relief. It relieves hoarseness and asthma without anxiety. When there is intestinal catarrh, painful and hot hemorrhoids, or a painful anus, ginger tea will help.

When the body doesn't digest protein easily and has produced too much acid, a slice of ginger root or a pinch of ginger powder in hot water can calm the body and digestive processes. Hot ginger tea stimulates a delayed menstrual period and relieves menstrual cramps.

Ginger has been used for relief of arthritis, rheumatism, sprains, muscular aches, and other pains. It is used for loss of appetite, chills, and infectious diseases such as colds and flu. It is helpful in relieving catarrh, congestion, sore throats, sinusitis, and coughs.

– Horseradish –

This plant is widely used in the southern part of Germany. It is given when frontal bones hurt, for sinus trouble, and for salivary gland difficulties. In this region, people gargle with horseradish broth if they have throat problems, hoarseness, or hearing problems.

Farmers use horseradish for cataracts and inflammation of the eyes. The root is grated and eaten raw or a broth is made. When there is a burning or cutting feeling in glands, which is worse at night, try horseradish. Horseradish boiled in apple juice gives copious urine if the kidney is blocked.

Horseradish is helpful in digestion. It is also used as a pain reliever for neck and back pain.

Horseradish is known to raise vital life forces.

– **Juniper** –

"A remedy to treat tapeworm: juniper berries 5 parts, white oil 5 parts, is taken for one day." Egyptian writings 1550 B.C.

This spice has been used in healing throughout history. In European folk medicine, juniper was used for dysentery, cholera, typhoid, tapeworm, and other ills of the poor. Juniper leaves are used for ridding the body of parasites.

Juniper berries are used to rid the body of toxins associated with arthritis and gout. They reduce indigestion, gas, and urinary infections. The tea is used for menstrual cramps or an upset stomach.

Juniper berries are a gentle stimulant and diuretic. They impart the smell of violets in the urine. They are extremely beneficial to the kidneys and help reduce tissue swelling.

– **Lemon Balm** –

"Balm, given every morning, will renew youth, strengthen the brain, and relieve languishing nature." London Dispensary 1696

Used medicinally by the Greeks 2,000 years ago, lemon balm was called "heart's delight."

Lemon balm has been used throughout history in preparations designed to promote youth. It was reputed to have been drunk every morning by Llewlyn, Prince of Glamorgan, who lived to be 108 years old. It is thought to strengthen the brain, aid depression, and it is used as a sedative.

Lemon balm helps indigestion, especially during worry or anxiety. It is antibacterial and antiviral in nature, probably because it contains tannins. It has been used to relieve nausea, flatulence, insomnia, and menstrual pain.

Lemon balm appears to deter colds and flu when taken at the onset of the illness. It has also been used for asthma and bronchitis. Steam inhalation of lemon balm tea relieves bronchial catarrh and sore throats. Lemon balm repels insects and is thought to relieve insect bites when applied externally.

~ Mace ~

Mace is the covering of nutmeg. If burned as incense, as the American Indians do, it increases a sense of self discipline and increases concentration power. For medicinal uses, please refer to nutmeg.

~ **Marjoram** ~

Marjoram has been used historically as a symbol of happiness and to give peace to departed spirits. Marjoram tea was recommended by the early herbalist, Gerard, for people who "are given to overmuch sighing."

Marjoram tea is a mild tonic which aids fever situations. Marjoram has been used for headaches, gastrointestinal difficulties, and nervous disorders. It can be calming to the respiratory system and assist in relieving migraines and muscle spasms.

Add marjoram tea or oil to the bath for relief of rheumatism and tension. Put a drop of marjoram oil on the pillow to induce sleep. Its aromatic influences are said to be peace, celibacy, and sleep.

To relieve a sore throat, soak a cotton cloth in marjoram tea and wrap it around the throat. Wrap another, larger cloth over it, making it as airtight as possible, and leave on several hours or overnight.

~ **Mustard Seed** ~

Mustard is such a fast growing plant that, in the past, it was said that you could grow the mustard greens for the salad for dinner while the meat was roasting. Mustard has been used to draw the blood to the surface of the skin or lungs and to relieve pain and inflammation in rheumatism, arthritis, chills, and congested lungs. Added to a foot bath, mustard warms and deodorizes the feet and relieves a cold.

Mustard is a blood purifier and a laxative. Swallow two mustard seeds a day to improve memory.

~ Myrrh ~

Myrrh is one of the spices brought to Jesus at His birth by the three kings of the Orient and has been considered a treasure of the East for thousands of years. Myrrh in lamb's blood was used by Moses on doors to help ward off the plague.

In Ancient Egypt, women burned myrrh to get rid of fleas in their homes. It has a particularly unpleasant taste but has been found to be excellent for sore throats and mouth ulcers. (Use as a gargle.)

Ancient Greeks used myrrh to heal wounds and it is used in chest rubs for congestion and bronchitis. Used as a tincture, it relieves infectious ailments like colds or glandular fever.

It has been found by the Arabic people to help skin conditions such as athlete's foot, eczema, cracked skin, ringworm, and wrinkles. It was also used for asthma, coughs, and bronchitis.

Myrrh seems to help mouth conditions such as gum infections, gingivitis, sore throats, and mouth ulcers. It may also be beneficial in digestive difficulties such as diarrhea, gas and indigestion and may aid hemorrhoids. It is thought to cleanse the prostate system and balance hypothyroid problems.

The whole plant is thought to be a useful tonic and the root is a valuable tonic for girls ages 15 to 18, as well as a strengthening tonic for the elderly.

~ **Myrtle** ~

Myrtle is used very little in cooking. Myrtle leaves contain Myrtal, an active antiseptic. It is used as a tea for bronchitis, coughing and cystitis and helps when there is thick, yellow mucous.

"Stitches" (or a quick, painful throbbing feeling) in the left breast always calls for myrtle. Myrtle is a nerve sedative, particularly when people are worse in the morning. Myrtle can be used as a tea for psoriasis and sinusitis and as a compress for bruises and hemorrhoids.

~ **Nutmeg** ~

Nutmeg has been used in China since the 7th century and was introduced to Europe by the Portuguese in 1512.

Nutmeg is my favorite spice. If given sparingly, it stops fainting fits. It helps in weak heartbeats. When one staggers when trying to walk, nutmeg provides an excellent service. Also, when people change from laughing and enjoyment to being bewildered and confused, nutmeg will help.

The most help is given when the digestive enzymes of the pancreas cannot reach the duodenum. The outlet is swollen and people complain of a swollen pancreas. Take 6 to 7 ounces of hot water and add 1 teaspoon of cloves and a dash of nutmeg (about 1/4 teaspoon). Drink this mixture and immediately the valve opens and there is no trouble anymore.

When the tongue adheres to the roof of the mouth, take nutmeg. When the abdomen is distended without nausea, try nutmeg. When objects appear distorted in size, use nutmeg.

Nutmeg has been found to be beneficial for boils and pimples. Take 1/3 teaspoon of nutmeg in 4 or 5 ounces of water with 1 teaspoon honey added. Drink this 3 mornings in a row. Then don't drink it for 3 days. Repeat this process 9 times.

Nutmeg is also useful for teen-agers because it makes them more self-reliant. Make them a nutmeg bath by adding 1 heaping teaspoon of nutmeg to a bathtub full of water and let them soak.

Nutmeg aids digestive problems and relieves nausea, vomiting, diarrhea, and food poisoning. Nutmeg oil can be applied to aching teeth with a cotton swab until dental treatment is available.

Nutmeg tea inspires sleep and is thought to overcome frigidity, impotence, and nervous fatigue. Use this spice sparingly because large doses can be poisonous and can cause a miscarriage.

~ **Oregano** ~

This delightful cooking and healing spice was named by the Greeks who called it *oros ganos* which means joy of the mountain. It is wild marjoram.

Aristotle reported that tortoises that ate a snake would immediately eat oregano to prevent death, so it was used as an antidote for poison at that time. Its aromatic influence is to strengthen the feeling of security.

Oregano has anti-viral qualities and may aid the body in balancing metabolism. It is useful as a tea for coughs, stomach and gallbladder problems, and menstrual pains.

Oregano has also been used for nervous headaches, irritability, exhaustion, and as a sedative. It is thought to prevent seasickness. It can be applied externally for swelling, rheumatism, and a stiff neck.

Chewing on an oregano leaf provides temporary relief for a toothache.

~ Parsley ~

Parsley was held in high esteem by the Greeks and was used to crown winners of games. The Greeks used parsley medicinally, although the Romans were the first known to use it as a food or spice. Parsley is rich in nutrients such as vitamins, minerals, and antiseptic chlorophyll.

Parsley can be chewed raw to freshen the breath and promote healthy skin. Eating parsley after garlic or onion will help deodorize the breath and the body.

Used as a tea, it is a digestive aid. Its use encourages free flow of urine. It can also be used as a poultice for insect bites and wounds. To soften hard breasts in the early stage of nursing, apply bruised parsley to the breasts.

People who have high blood pressure or arthritis should eat plenty of raw parsley in salads. Parsley is a good food to keep the arteries clear.

For bladder stones or kidney stones, drink 1 quart of parsley tea a day for 3 days and then just 2 cups a day. Another recipe is to drink parsley tea for 3 days with no other food for these stones.

For loose teeth, drink 3 cups of parsley tea a day.

Parsley root has been used as a natural diuretic and to benefit kidney conditions. It is also a mild laxative.

– **Peppermint** –

"If any man can name . . . all the properties of mint, he must know how many fish swim in the Indian Ocean." Wilafried of Strabo 12th century

Peppermint is a favorite beverage tea all over the world. It elevates and opens the sensory system. It has been found to be very purifying and stimulating to the mind as well as the body.

Peppermint is well known to help indigestion, intestinal spasms, gas, colic, and other similar conditions, particularly in children. Peppermint stimulates the liver. Peppermint leaves in cottage cheese taste good and helps digestion.

Peppermint aids nausea and travel sickness and is helpful for fever and flu. It is analgesic, calming, and good for headaches and migraines.

Peppermint is used to soothe sore throats and is antibacterial. For sinus problems, drink lots of peppermint tea and apply a large, warm peppermint pack to the sinus area for immediate relief.

If every scratch becomes a sore, peppermint tea is helpful. It can be used as an eyewash for inflammations and as a wash for skin ailments, itching, burns, ringworm, and bug bites.

Peppermint can be used for shingles, as well as infected or painful nerves. For vaginal itching, use a very mild tea of peppermint as a douche to bring relief.

If one of your loved ones has to have an operation, place peppermint leaves on their picture and pray for healing. The operation will have no side effects and the healing time will be shorter with no complications.

~ **Rosemary** ~

"Rosemary is for remembrance. . ."

Shakespeare

The Spanish revered rosemary as the bush that sheltered the Virgin Mary on her flight to Egypt. As she spread her cloak over the herb, the white flowers turned blue.

This spice has a long history of medicinal and culinary uses and was thought to improve memory and promote fidelity. It was introduced to Europe around the 14th century. Rosemary is an excellent tonic and is thought to promote youthfulness. It is uplifting, energizing, and helpful for headaches and depression.

In early times, rosemary was burned in sickrooms to purify the air. During the plague of 1665, it was carried by individuals to sniff occasionally to ward off the disease. John Gerard mentions rosemary as a breath freshener. He advises that eating the flower every morning with bread and salt, "it helps dim eyes, and procures a clear sight."

Rosemary is known as a blood thinner and strengthens heart muscles and weak stomachs. It is helpful for colds and flu and is known to help digestive difficulties. Rosemary stimulates circulation and eases pain by increasing the flow of blood where applied. It aids in fat digestion and is used for aching joints and rheumatism.

Rosemary has been used to stimulate delayed menses, prevent miscarriage, and is restorative to the female system. It has also been used for nervous upsets, headaches, exhaustion, and for congestion of the liver.

It may encourage the immune system and is thought to improve candida conditions. Having rosemary tea every morning is thought to have restorative qualities and "comfort the brain." A sprig of rosemary under the pillow has been known to alleviate children's nightmares.

The tea makes an excellent hair rinse, encouraging growth, relieving dandruff, and restoring color. It also makes an excellent antiseptic mouthwash and gargle.

~ Sage ~

"How can a man grow old who has sage in his garden?" Ancient Chinese Proverb

The name *salvia* is the Latin word for sage and means good health, to cure, and to save. Both in early Roman culture and American Indian culture, sage has been considered a sacred spice.

The American Indians used sage tea to rub down the body and in a bath to reduce fevers.

Sage has long been considered an aid to failing memory, especially in the elderly, and has been associated with helping people to live long lives. Make a sandwich by putting sage on buttered bread. It is very delicious. Sage is known as a food for the brain, as well as an antidepressant. This is also known to relieve allergies.

Sage is an excellent tonic, liver stimulant, and improves digestive function. Sage tea helps the body digest proteins and helps the body and nervous system relax. It is antiseptic, anti-fungal, and contains natural estrogen.

Sage has an affinity to the mouth and is often used as a mouthwash and gargle to help sore throats, gum disease, and mouth ulcers. It is also thought to prevent the graying of the hair.

Sage tea can be used as an antiseptic by pouring the tea on a pad and applying to the skin to help slow healing wounds. It is excellent for reducing the secretions of the body and has been found beneficial in reducing salivation in Parkinson's disease. It is good for night sweats, vaginal discharge, excessive perspiration, and to slow the flow of milk. It is a uterine stimulant, reduces blood sugar, and promotes the flow of bile.

Use sage for glandular weakness and bloated conditions. For vericose veins or ulcers on the legs, apply hot sage compresses. Use sage tea on the leg and take frequent sage foot baths. Sage is also thought to improve a weak spine. ⌒

– **Savory** –

Savory is a spice which has a flavor similar to pepper. It stimulates the mental body and the adrenal cortex. It is considered an antiseptic and is beneficial to the whole digestive tract. It stimulates the appetite, eases indigestion and flatulence, and can be used as a tonic. It is good for gastric pains of nervous origin.

Savory tea has been used as an antiseptic mouthwash and gargle. It has been used in mental and sexual debility. In Germany, it is used for all types of diarrhea and has been known to rid the body of intestinal parasites. It has been known to help some types of deafness. Savory is antibacterial, anti-fungal, and anti-viral and has been used to treat staph and candida. ⌒

– **Thyme** –

Thyme is one of the herbs blessed with a large number of therapeutic properties. The origin of the name thyme may be the Greek word *thymon*, which means courage, and many of the early uses of this spice were to enhance that virtue. Roman soldiers bathed in thyme water to improve their vigor.

Romans also used thyme to repel insects and scorpions and for snake bites and the bites of marine creatures. Scottish Highlanders drank thyme tea for strength and courage, as well as to prevent nightmares. It has also been used to overcome shyness and to stimulate intelligence.

In early medicine, thyme was so important for its use for female disorders that it was often called "mother." It seems to have an affinity to the uterus and has been used to relieve menstrual pain and restore balance during abnormal absence of menstrual periods.

Thyme is antibacterial, anti-parasitic, and antiseptic in nature. It stimulates the production of white blood cells to aid the body in resisting infection. It is thought to help the body resist colds and flu. Thyme tea with honey relieves illness resulting from chill such as coughs, colds, flu, sore throats, and postnasal drip. It has been used for asthma, tuberculosis, and other bronchial disorders such as emphysema and mycosis (lung fungus).

Thyme tea relieves insomnia, fatigue, and other mental debilities such as anxiety and depression.

It relieves muscular pain and improves capillary circulation.

Thyme is a digestive tonic, improves sluggish digestion, and can be used to detoxify from a hangover. It has been used for gastric problems such as colic, indigestion, gas, irritable bowels, and bad breath. It has been used to treat parasites such as roundworm, tapeworm, threadworm, and hookworm.

Thyme tea is a reliable folk remedy for relieving phlegm and shortness of breath. It has been used as a skin antiseptic for lice, scabies, insect bites, and snake bites. It heals wounds quickly. It is also found to be helpful to prevent or stop hair loss.

Culpepper says, "It is so harmless you need not fear the use of it."

~ Turmeric ~

Recently it was found that turmeric contains a substance which significantly reduces the long-term recurrence of viruses. It also halts tumor growth. Just use a small amount.

Section II: Additional Kitchen Remedies

~ Almond ~

Almonds are a good brain tonic. Almond oil, only 1 teaspoon daily, will improve your memory. Almonds contain natural Laetrile, or vitamin B17, which helps counteract cancer. ~

~ Apple ~

"An apple a day keeps the doctor away."
Early American adage

The apple is the queen of all fruits. It is a universal food, which means it can be eaten with anything without causing indigestion.

Apples are a tonic for the body and are a stimulant for the liver and digestive system. They have both a laxative effect and a diuretic effect on the body. Apples seem to be beneficial to fevers and colds. A mixture of apple juice and olive oil has been used as an antiseptic for cuts and abrasions.

From France comes this good news: an apple a day can lower cholesterol. This was reported in the *Medical Tribune.*

The whole apple is balm to the gallbladder. Dried apple peelings made into a tea are full of silicon and will strengthen muscles, improve other kinds of weaknesses, and are good for rheumatic fever.

Apples agree with most people. Raw and finely grated, apples will stop your child's diarrhea.

Apple juice is excellent and can soften gall-stones and kidney stones.

Make a tea of apple tree bark and drink it warm. It will check miscarriages. ⤢

– **Apple Cider Vinegar** –

Combat food poisoning with apple cider vinegar. Take 2 teaspoons of apple cider vinegar in 7 ounces of warm water and sip slowly. For children, add honey.

For parasites: keep parasites out of your body by taking 2 teaspoons of apple cider vinegar every day in 6 to 7 ounces of water. If you travel overseas, take apple cider vinegar with you and take it twice a day.

Interestingly, taking apple cider vinegar every

day also keeps mosquitoes from biting you. They will land and then take off without biting.

For asthma: soak two pieces of cloth in apple cider vinegar and wrap around each wrist. Secure with Saran Wrap. Very good! ⤨

~ **Apricot** ~

Apricots with their kernels, plus calcium carbonate (lime), are your best foods for natural Laetrile. You can also use peach seeds, almonds, or millet.

Here is the recipe for your homemade B17:

- 4 apricot kernels
- 2 pieces dried apricots
- 5 Calcerea Carb. 6X homeopathic or limewater

Chew this together. Take the formula twice a day. It tastes wonderful. Everybody should have this treat at least once a day! ⤨

~ **Arrowroot** ~

This is a food for the weak, debilitated, and those who are convalescing. It is very easily digested, creating no gastric upset.

People who suffer from bacterial dysentery or gastric upset would find it most suitable. Take 1 teaspoon of arrowroot, make a smooth paste with cold milk or water, stir well, and boil. Add a little lime juice just before you take it.

~ Artichoke ~

Artichokes tone up the liver. They bring clear urine and increase the flow of bile. Artichokes are thought to help keep arteries clean and smooth and improve weak digestion. It is useful for albumin in the urine and jaundice.

~ Asparagus ~

Asparagus is a wonderful diuretic. It is cooling, soothing, and a tremendous addition to any diet, especially when tumors are present. Take 4 tablespoons asparagus twice a day for cancerous conditions. Asparagus is also known to dissolve kidney stones.

Asparagus contains substances that assist the body in normal cell formation. Asparagus contains a great deal of iodine and may be helpful in preventing cancer and other cell destroying diseases.

– **Banana** –

Bananas are loaded with potassium. We need potassium to keep our heart in order, to help keep bones healthy, and to keep the blood and lymph systems fit.

Lack of potassium is known to cause leg cramps, especially at night. Before you take potassium pills, ask yourself how much fruit you are eating. Because of the potassium content, bananas can also balance excess water in the system and are good to relieve waterlogged tissues.

Bananas help combat heartburn and they are a bulk producer. They are also used for colitis, leukorrhea, backache, and as a diuretic.

DON'T eat bananas if you have a cold or cough, as they will add to the problems. You can make a compress for swollen tonsils with banana baked in the skin, mashed with a little fresh cream or olive oil.

– **Barley** –

Barley is an excellent food for children suffering from diarrhea or other inflammation of the bowels.

~ Beet ~

Red beets are good for anemia, leukemia, low blood sugar, stomach ailments, and septic blood. The lymph system and the spleen greatly benefit from beets.

Beets are high in potassium. Research at the University of Minnesota revealed that beets have an anti-carcinogenic hormone.

~ Cabbage ~

Cabbage has been called the medicine of the poor and is extremely valuable for its healing qualities. Research indicates that cabbage contains ingredients which prevent cancer, making it an important addition to any diet.

It is anti-inflammatory, antibacterial, and encourages new cell growth. It is helpful for digestive problems and lung problems. Cabbage improves hair, bones, and teeth.

It helps kidney disorders and heart problems. Cabbage is also helpful in hyperacidity and gastric ulcers. It has been used for headaches, aches and pains, and fluid retention,

Shredded cabbage is terrific as a poultice for swollen knees, ankles, or elbows. Wrap shredded cabbage in a clean cloth and apply overnight to the swollen joint. Repeat this process several nights in a row for best results. ❧

— **Carrot** —

Carrots are great for maintaining good health and are one of the foods mentioned with regard to the life-giving properties of Rhodium and Iridium.

It is a blood builder and contains vitamins A and C. Carrots are good for eyesight and help prevent night blindness. Cooked carrots relieve stomach ulcers.

For canker sores: wrap finely grated carrot with cloth and lay against the canker sore. Change every 2 hours. ❧

— **Cherry** —

Sour cherries are a good remedy for gout by eating 1 small dish of sour cherries every morning for 3 weeks. Eat cherries morning and night for hypochondria. Cherry juice is good for people who urinate constantly. A glass of cherry juice 3 or 4 times a day will relieve this situation. ❧

~ **Coconut** ~

Coconut is a natural diuretic and it purifies the blood. It nourishes the prostate gland and the testicles and removes heat or burning sensation from these organs. It is useful for women to reduce the flow of menses. It is a tonic for the kidneys and is useful for hyperacidity.

Pregnant women should drink coconut water in the morning on an empty stomach. It will bring clear urine and will greatly nourish the fetus.

Coconut oil is excellent for massage. It is used for skin disorders such as itching, eczema, and dermatitis.

The following is a treatment for cataracts in the eyes: take fresh coconut juice and, with an eye dropper, apply as much as the eye can hold. Apply hot wet cloths for about 10 minutes while lying down. Several treatments are needed.

Coconut is food for the brain. I know of one student at the University of Freiburg. He was not too bright and studied many hours while the rest of his colleagues went swimming and were having fun. All this changed when his uncle sent him coconuts. He drank the milk and ate the meat and soon he was as bright as the others.

~ **Cranberry Juice** ~

Use concentrated cranberry juice for asthma. When an asthma attack is imminent, put 1/2 teaspoon or less of the cranberry concentrate on the inside of the bottom lip. Use only a small amount so that the person will not choke. This might snap the person out of the attack immediately.

Cranberry juice should be drunk on a regular basis by people suffering from asthma, as well as from kidney and bladder disorders.

~ **Cucumber** ~

Cucumbers are a delightful vegetable with many medicinal uses. Cucumbers are very good for the skin, especially the complexion. Either eaten or used topically, they cool and heal the skin.

Cucumber satisfies thirst and it is a very good diuretic. Cucumber contains a hormone needed by the pancreas for insulin production. Its natural sodium makes stiff joints more limber. It reduces the intoxicating effect of alcohol.

Cucumber juice purifies the lymphatic system, cleans the blood, and relieves jaundice. Drink 4 or 5 cups of freshly pressed cucumber juice for this cleansing process.

~ Egg ~

Egg yolk mixed in concord grape juice is an excellent blood builder. Egg white, slightly beaten, applied to first and second degree burns will relieve the pain immediately.

~ Eggplant ~

Eggplant stimulates the appetite. It is food for the spleen. Eat 2 to 3 small pieces of cooked eggplant before breakfast on an empty stomach to reduce an enlarged spleen.

Eggplant increases red blood cells, improving anemia. It is also known as a good tonic. If eggplant is sliced and placed in lightly salted water for about 20 minutes, the bitter taste will be alleviated.

Eggplant skin is very important in the treatment of tumors. Peel the eggplant 1/2 inch thick (leaving on 1/2 inch of the meat). Boil, steam, or broil these peelings until soft. Season with kelp or dulse. This remedy relieves tumors and cellulite. Enjoy it!

~ Elderberry Juice ~

Elderberry juice is terrific for sciatica and facial twitching.

– Epsom Salts –

Epsom salts are useful to relieve pain in the hands and feet, especially after a sprain or with arthritis. Put about 1 tablespoon of Epsom salts in warm water and soak for about 20 minutes.

For facial pimples: make a mask of Epsom salts and water and pat on the afflicted area with cotton before going to bed. Do this every night until pimples are gone.

For shingles: make a paste of Epsom salts and water and pat on the afflicted area with cotton. Relief should come in a short time.

– Grapefruit –

Eating grapefruit is helpful if you have ringing in the ears or other head noises. Try eating a piece of grapefruit if you have pain in the temporal region.

– Honey –

We call honey "the ambrosia of the gods." Each area within a country has its own distinctive type of honey. It is said that, to relieve allergy symptoms, use honey from your own neighborhood. It can act as an antihistamine.

Put honey on sores and they will heal quickly. It is antiseptic and antibacterial. During war shortages, honey was often used with oil or lard as a dressing for small wounds or ulcers. It was so used in Shanghai during World War II.

The simple sugars in honey are quickly absorbed by the body, so it can give you a quick lift when needed. Add water or tea to honey and drink it. In early history, Olympic athletes ate great quantities of honey before the games in preparation for the events. This is still done today.

Apple cider vinegar, honey, and water, together, have been used for thousands of years by many different cultures to "balance" the body. This combination has also been found to be extremely beneficial to people with gout or arthritic pain when taken every morning. It has been known to restore supple movement in hands and dissolve knots.

Honey can also be beneficial for respiratory problems and relieves cough and sore throats. For fever, drink hot lemon juice with honey.

– **Lemon** –

Use lemon peel for calluses, corns, or warts. Put the lemon peel (white side down) on afflicted area and cover with a Band-Aid to hold it in place overnight. Every night put on a fresh piece.

~ **Lettuce** ~

Lettuce, like spinach, is rich in vitamins A, B, C, and E. It stimulates the smooth operation of the digestive tract and adds needed bulk to the diet.

Lettuce water is an excellent remedy for a virus infection. Take leaf lettuce and boil in water. Drink 4 ounces every hour.

Lettuce water can be applied externally over swollen parts of the body such as ankles, abdomen, and liver.

~ **Oats** ~

Found in most kitchens, oats can be helpful in our quest for health and well being. They are known to be a helpful tonic to the entire body and are thought to relieve depression and nervous disorders.

Oats are rich in silicon. They stimulate sweating and are helpful to the thyroid and for estrogen deficiency. They have been found to be helpful to reduce morphine addiction.

Oats have been used for degenerative conditions such as multiple sclerosis. An effective skin treatment, oats can be cooked in water and drained and the "oat water" can be added to the bath for relief from shingles, eczema, herpes sores, and the itching of chicken pox.

Feeding oatmeal to children is said to stimulate their appetite, which can be useful when a child is not flourishing. Oatmeal is also extremely healing internally and may be used by any invalid during any convalescence.

It is used in the Bach Flower Remedies in times of uncertainty and dissatisfaction. Sleeping on a mattress of oat straw is thought to heal bones and straighten out a curved spine.

~ **Okra** ~

Okra has many healing properties and it has been said that "eating okra will heal anything." Okra is especially useful as a general tonic for the body and has been found useful in cases of heavy menstrual bleeding.

~ **Onion** ~

Onions have always been known to have antibacterial properties. Since onions easily absorb bacteria, they can be used in a sickroom to help disinfect it.

Onion broth is restorative. Onion increase the circulation and stimulates and warms the body. If you are sensitive to light, increase your use of red onion. It is also used for neuralgia pain and it helps chronic neuritis. It is a blessing for long-standing ulcers on heels.

For ear problems such as a recurring ear infection or ringing in the ear, cut a yellow onion in half and rub on the back of the ear. For a splinter, rub onion on the area.

For hay fever, cough, a tickling larynx, or an oncoming flu, sip on red onion soup. Soup recipe: take several red onions and break them up. INCLUDE the papery skin. Simmer in water for about 20 minutes and strain. Sip on a little of this broth every hour until relief is obtained.

~ **Orange** ~

The orange originally came from China where it has long been used as a medicine. If you have a headache with nausea or facial neuralgia mostly right-sided, try an orange. Peel it and eat 1/2 orange.

For hiccups, a never-fail recipe is to take an orange and cut it in half. Squeeze the juice from 1/2 of the orange into a glass and drink it slowly. If needed, do the same to the other half.

Oranges are used as a digestive remedy, aiding in the treatment of constipation. Try boiled orange peels if you are constipated. It increases the bile for hours.

In the Old Country, dried boiled orange peelings are used for cancer patients having pain, particularly if the cancer is in the mouth or tongue. This recipe is also used to stop female hemorrhages.

Eating oranges helps relieve thick mucous-type coughing and is thought to relieve and prevent colds. It calms the nerves and is useful for depression, insomnia, and shock.

– Pear –

Cut pears into small pieces and eat a piece every 15 minutes all day to relieve the kidney of mucous and accumulated poisons.

– Pineapple –

Pineapple juice is a good source of vitamin C and can be used as a remedy for hiccups.

– Pomegranate –

Pomegranate is used to expel tapeworm. If you are constantly hungry or feel "jumpy" and nervous inside, a little pomegranate will stabilize this condition. ⌒

– **Pumpkin** –

Pumpkin is high in beta carotene and is, therefore, an excellent food. It calms an upset stomach. Pumpkin seeds are used to rid the body of parasites. Pumpkin seed tea is used for gallbladder troubles. To make the tea, take 1 teaspoon of ground pumpkin seeds, pour 1 cup of hot water over them, and let it steep for a few minutes. Drink 2 cups of tea a day. ⌒

– **Salt** –

For pain, heat salt in a frying pan. Fill a cloth sack with the heated salt and place over the painful area. Cover with a hot water bottle to keep it warm. It's amazing how well this inexpensive trick works.

For rattlesnake bite, wet some salt and wrap the bitten arm or leg in a salt pack, making sure the bite gets an extra dose of salt. Then rush to your physician. ⌒

~ **Sesame Seed** ~

Sesame seeds prevent nervous breakdown and promote a strong will in people. Sesame seed supplies osmium, a trace mineral.

It is also a food for the glands and is a supplier of complete amino acids. Sesame seeds relieve constipation, hemorrhoids, and genitourinary infections.

~ **Sunflower Seed** ~

Sunflower seeds are very helpful for eyestrain and sensitivity to light. Even aches and pains disappear when you nibble about 1/2 cup of seeds a day.

~ **Tomato** ~

Always cut the place out which was attached to the vine. This is nightshade poison and, when removed, the tomato is a fabulous food and remedy for well and sick days. Tomatoes, including tomato juice, contain lycopene which is a substance known to reduce tumors.

A slice of tomato on swelling reduces it quickly. A young man had such swollen glands due to mononucleosis that he was about to have an operation. His father applied raw tomato poultices to the neck and all swelling left in 2 hours. Raw tomatoes can also be applied to the head in cases of brain tumors.

Stewed tomatoes will cleanse the pancreas when combined with lime and will assist in the digestion of proteins. Apply mashed ripe tomatoes to the soles of your feet when they are painful and leave it on overnight. The next morning, all pain will be gone.

~ **Wheat Sprouts** ~

Wheat sprouts will improve detoxification of tissue and protect against heavy metal damage in the body.

~ **Yam** ~

Yam was used in the original contraceptive pills because it contains substances very similar to progesterone. It appears to be beneficial to menopausal women.

It has also been called colic root for its soothing properties in colic conditions. It is a tonic for the spleen and stomach and has been used for ailments of the kidneys, lung, and stomach, as well as urinary infections and asthma.

The following are items commonly found in the kitchen which can be very beneficial in health and wellness. ⌒

Latest Research

There has been recent research which indicates that two trace minerals are extremely important to our health and well being. These two trace minerals, when included in the diet, can greatly enhance our life force, health, and vitality. **They are Iridium and Rhodium and are superconductors of spiritual light.** Foods which contain both of these trace minerals are listed below with the ratio of the trace minerals present in them:

Essiac Tea	60 Rhodium 10 Iridium
Concord Grape Juice	120 Rhodium 48 Iridium
Fresh Carrot Juice	15 Rhodium 15 Iridium
Watercress	27 Rhodium 35 Iridium
Aloe Vera	37 Rhodium 7 Iridium

St. John's Wort   7 Rhodium
                           6 Iridium

Shark Oil   13 Rhodium
                           2 Iridium

It is obvious that, to ensure the vitality of your life force, it is advisable to use these foods every day. One half cup of concord grape juice or fresh carrot juice will be enough.

Further research has discovered that concord grape juice can be used to combat cancer in the following way: every morning for 6 weeks, drink 1 quart of concord grape juice from the time you wake up until noon, with no other food during that time. After noon, begin eating normally. You should emphasize almonds, asparagus, and other fruits and vegetables and have no meat protein after 2 P.M.

Rhodium and Iridium are available in homeopathic form at Hanna's Herb Shop (303-443-0755). Ask for the product: "Life Center."

SPICES TO THE RESCUE

Hanna speaks of coming from a missionary family: "My parents taught us to help in a simple way. Mother had the natural gift of healing and father, a chemist, supported her with a knowledge of chemistry so her natural healing was really based on chemical knowledge."

"Often we do not have the chemicals on hand but we can go to our kitchen and look in our spice cabinet and at our foods, which are common in all households."

"We are living in a time of a health crisis and I support the knowledge of my parents and bring it to your house."

SPICES TO THE RESCUE

Books by Hanna

"Wholistic health represents an attitude toward well being which recognizes that we are not just a collection of mechanical parts, but an integrated system which is physical, mental, social and spiritual."

Ageless Remedies from Mother's Kitchen
You will laugh and be amazed at all that you can do in your own pharmacy, the kitchen. These time tested treasures are in an easy to read, cross referenced guide. (94 pages)

Allergy Baking Recipes
Easy and tasty recipes for cookies, cakes, muffins, pancakes, breads and pie crusts. Includes wheat free recipes, egg and milk free recipes (and combinations thereof) and egg and milk substitutes. (34 pages)

Alzheimer's Science and God
This little booklet provides a closer look at this disease and presents Hanna's unique, religious perspectives on Alzheimer's disease. (15 pages)

Arteriosclerosis and Herbal Chelation
A booklet containing information on Arteriosclerosis causes, symptoms and herbal remedies. An introduction to the product *Circu Flow*. (17 pages)

Cancer: Traditional and New Concepts
A fascinating and extremely valuable collection of theories, tests, herbal formulas and special information pertaining to many facets of this dreaded disease. (65 pages)

Cookbook for Electro-Chemical Energies
The opening of this book describes basic principles of healthy eating along with some fascinating facts you may not have heard before. The rest of this book is loaded with delicious, healthy recipes. A great value. (106 pages)

God Helps Those That Help Themselves
This work is a beautifully comprehensive description of the seven basic physical causes of disease. It is wholistic information as we need it now. A truly valuable volume. (270 pages)

Good Health Through Special Diets
This book shows detailed outlines of different diets for different needs. Dr. Reidlin, M.D. said, "The road to health goes through the kitchen not through the drug store," and that's what this book is all about. (121 pages)

Hanna's Workshops
A workbook that brings together all of the tools for applying Hanna's testing methods. Designed with 60 templates that enable immediate results.

How to Counteract Environmental Poisons
A wonderful collection of notes and information gleaned from many years of Hanna's teachings. This concise and valuable book discusses many toxic materials in our environment and shows you how to protect yourself from them. It also presents Hanna's insights on how to protect yourself, your family and your community from spiritual dangers. (53 pages)

Instant Herbal Locator
This is the herbal book for the do-it-yourself person. This book is an easy cross referenced guide listing complaints and the herbs that do the job. Very helpful to have on hand. (122 pages)

Instant Vitamin-Mineral Locator
A handy, comprehensive guide to the nutritive values of vitamins and minerals. Used to determine bodily deficiencies of these essential elements and combinations thereof, and what to do about these deficiencies. According to your symptoms, locate your vitamin and mineral needs. A very helpful guide. (55 pages)

New Dimensions in Healing Yourself
The consummate collection of Hanna's teachings. An unequated volume that compliments all of her other books as well as her years of teaching. (155 pages)

Old Time Remedies for Modern Ailments
A collection of natural remedies from Eastern and Western cultures. There are 20 fast cleansing methods and many ways to rebuild your health. A health classic. (115 pages)

Parasites: The Enemy Within
A compilation of years of Hanna's studies with parasites. A rare treasure and one of the efforts to expose the truths that face us every day. (62 pages)

The Pendulum, the Bible and Your Survival
A guide booklet for learning to use a pendulum. Explains various aspects of energies, vibrations and forces. (22 pages)

The Seven Spiritual Causes of Ill Health
This book beautifully reveals how our spiritual and emotional states have a profound effect on our physical well being. It addresses fascinating topics such as karma, gratitude, trauma, laughter as medicine...and so much more. A wonderful volume full of timeless treasures. (145 pages)